KEEP CALM
AND STRETCH

Keep Calm and Stretch:
44 Stretching Exercises
To Increase Flexibility, Relieve Pain,
Prevent Injury, And Stay Young!

By: Julie Schoen

CONTENTS

INTRODUCTION

It is no secret that I am addicted to stretching. I stretch *all* the time – while I'm watching a movie, driving, writing, cooking, shopping, standing in line – you name it and I stretch while I am doing it. And while you might see me and think I'm crazy for stretching with my shopping cart as I peruse the produce, there is a reason behind my madness.

It feels *so* good.

I wasn't always into stretching. In fact I hated it. Even as an athlete I didn't see the point in it, so I would skip out on stretching sessions before and after I ran. I only started stretching after major injuries to my back forced me into it. Stretching, I learned, was the only way to relieve the intense pain I was experiencing. So although I was no good at it (I literally couldn't move), I started stretching on a daily basis. I was blown away at how good even the subtlest stretches felt. Soon, thanks to stretching, I was back to my good old self.

For me, my love of stretching turned into a love of yoga. When people asked me how I recovered from my own injuries and what I could recommend for them so that they could start feeling better too, I found myself always talking about yoga – yoga, yoga, and more yoga.

Unfortunately, not everyone shares my love of yoga. In fact, some people, maybe even you, have a downright disdain for it. And that's okay. I'll be the first to admit that it is not for everyone. But, what is for everyone is stretching. Everyone can do it anywhere they want and they don't need anything. Stretching is universally awesome.

So regardless of your current body or state of mind, I guarantee you that after a bit of stretching you will feel a million times better. It always works.

Keep Calm and Stretch On!

Love,

Julie

WHY IS STRETCHING GOOD FOR ME?

Stretching is one of the most overlooked solutions for many of the ailments that are byproducts of our modern lifestyles. Just by stretching every day you are ridding the body of pain, keeping the body feeling young and healthy, preventing injuries, healing injuries, and managing stress.

Here are the top 10 reasons for why you should start stretching – now!

1. Stretching increases flexibility and range of motion in the body so you can stay active
2. Stretching increases the amount of energy you have
3. Stretching relieves pain in the body, including pain you may have been dealing with for years and years
4. Stretching prevents injuries by keeping the muscles flexible and long

5. Because your circulation improves and increases when you stretch, stretching helps to heal injuries – fast
6. Stretching helps to improve muscle coordination and balance, preventing injuries that could be caused by falling
7. Many stretches help to relieve pain in the lower back by increasing the flexibility of the hamstrings, hips, and gluteus muscles
8. Stretching lowers blood pressure
9. Stretching helps to relieve tension in the body which translates to less tension and stress in your life
10. Stretching improves your posture which helps to keep you looking confident and lean

WHY AM I NOT GETTING MORE FLEXIBLE?

There is a common complaint heard among people who have been consistently stretching for weeks, maybe even months, and that is: I am not getting any more flexible!

And while there are many reasons that can explain this frustrating phenomenon, including improper form and stretching only large muscle groups over and over again, one of the most common explanations is that you are not practicing stretching *with* resistance.

Resistance is key to getting more flexible. In fact, it is impossible to make progress stretching if you are not doing it. Resistance, although it may seem counterintuitive, actually helps to lengthen the muscles by contracting opposing muscles. For example, if you want to increase the flexibility of your hamstrings, you will hit a wall if you are not simultaneously increasing the resistance of the quadriceps. For this reason when I work with yoga students that have very stiff hamstrings, I encourage them to engage the quadriceps by lifting the kneecap as they stretch forward.

Contracting the opposing muscles actually helps you to lengthen the muscle you are targeting!

Another facet of stretching with resistance is that you want to find balance between pushing and pulling. You actually make more progress in improving flexibility by opposing the stretch. For example, when performing a simple shoulder stretch by bringing the arm across the body, you want to not just pull your arm forward, but you want to oppose the stretch with resistance by pressing your arm away from the body at the same time.

Any time you are using a body part, such as a hand or foot, to intensify the stretch, it is crucial to resist that body part by pressing into it with whatever is being stretched. This is the only way that you will start to see major improvements in your flexibility.

WHAT ARE THE BEST STRETCHES FOR MY BODY?

The best stretches are the ones that challenge your body, strengthening muscles while the opposing muscles are stretching. The following stretches are powerful because of their ability to adapt to a wide-range of bodies and capabilities, making them accessible and beneficial for everyone, no matter their starting point. **This series of stretches will allow you to increase flexibility in every major muscle group of the body, while also working into smaller groups that are often overlooked in basic stretches.**

Each stretch can be done on its own and before or after exercising. This series of stretches has also been designed so that you can work through them from start to finish for a total body stretch that will leave you feeling open, free from pain, and relaxed.

Elbow Behind Head

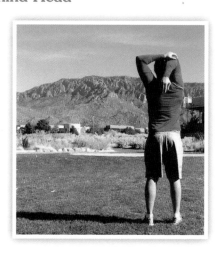

■ **Benefits:**

Stretches and increases the range of motion of the shoulders, a common site of stiffness and chronic pain.

■ **How-To:**

Standing tall, lift one arm straight into the air with the palm of the hand facing back. Place the hand on your upper back while using the other hand to gently pull your elbow closer towards the center of your head. Find a balance between pressing your elbow down and lifting the elbow up so as to create resistance as you stretch. As your range of motion increases, you can start to move the hand further down your back or try the bound stretch below.

Elbow Behind Head Bind

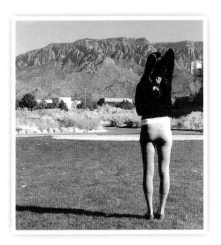

■ Benefits:

An intensified version of the regular Elbow Behind Head stretch, it will continue to create flexibility in your shoulders.

■ How-To:

Standing tall, lift one arm straight into the air with the palm of the hand facing back. Place the hand on your upper back while using the other hand to gently pull your elbow closer towards the center of your head. Then take the free arm down by your side, bending the elbow and sliding the top of your hand up the center of your back until you find your other hand. Clasp the fingers together. Stretch the chest open and pull the hands away from each other to maximize the benefits.

Twisted Wrist Roll

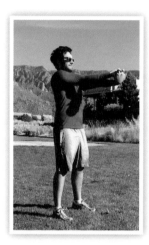 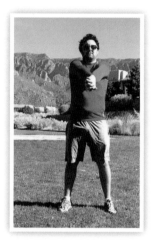

■ Benefits:

Stretches and rejuvenates the wrists. It is great for relieving and preventing pain caused by Carpal Tunnel Syndrome and other aches caused by repetitive motions such as typing.

■ How-To:

Stand up tall with your arms extended out in front of you, palms facing out. Cross one arm over the other and interlace the fingers. Roll the hands in towards your body and all the way through so that your arms are once again fully extended in front of you. Do your best to keep the chest open and the neck relaxed as you perform this stretch.

Wide Legged Forward Fold

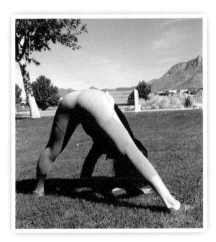

■ Benefits:

Stretches the hamstrings and inner thighs while lengthening the spine and loosening the muscles of the shoulders and neck. It is also great for relieving stress.

■ How-To:

Stand with your legs wide apart and feet parallel to each other. Squeeze the shoulder blades together to keep the back straight as you bend forward from the hips. When you have gone as low as you comfortably can, release the neck, shoulders, and back so that they can lengthen and relax. Bring your hands down under the shoulders or grab onto the outsides of your feet. To increase flexibility and strength, keep the fronts of the legs engaged by lifting the kneecaps.

Wide Legged Twist

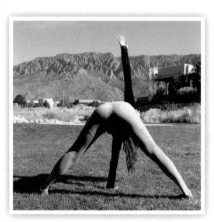

■ Benefits:

This stretch has all of the benefits of the Wide Legged Forward Fold with a gentle twist to help increase flexibility of the spine and rejuvenate and detoxify internal organs.

■ How-To:

Stand with your legs wide apart and feet parallel to each other. Squeeze the shoulder blades together to keep the back straight as you bend forward from the hips. When you have gone as low as you comfortably can, release the neck, shoulders, and back so that they can lengthen and relax. Bring your hands down under the shoulders. Leave one hand down on the ground while you extend the other arm up into the air, twisting from the hips. Try to get both arms in one straight line by simultaneously pushing the bottom arm forward and the top arm back.

Wide Legged Forward Bend With Clasp

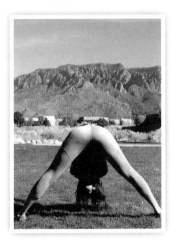 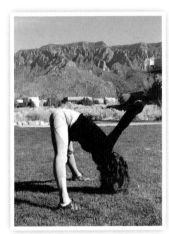

■ **Benefits:**

Stretches the hamstrings and inner thighs while calming the mind and cooling the body. The clasped hands open the shoulders and promote flexibility.

■ **How-To:**

Stand with your legs wide and feet parallel to each other. Fold forward keeping your back and legs as straight as possible. Then interlace the hands behind the back. Straighten the arms and let the hands fall over your head as much as possible. Keep the neck relaxed as you stretch.

Wide Legged Lunge

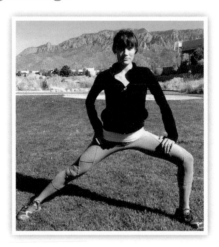

■ **Benefits:**

Stretches the inner thigh and groin muscles, helping to prevent injury while relieving tension in the lower back.

■ **How-To:**

Stand with your legs wide apart and feet parallel to each other. Bend one knee so that you lower into a side lunge keeping the bent knee right over the ankle. For a deeper stretch increase the distance between your feet.

Compass Twist

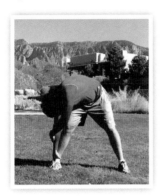 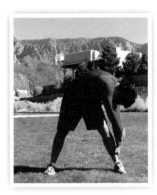

■ **Benefits:**

Stretches the backs of the legs and the side body, including the shoulder. The side-to-side motion in this stretch helps to increase range of motion while also strengthening small muscles of the back and the outer muscles of the abdomen.

■ **How-To:**

Stand with your legs slightly wider than your hips. Fold down and reach for one of your feet. If you cannot reach your foot without bending the knees, it is fine to place your hands on your shin or even your thigh. To create a stretch in the side body and outer shoulder, bring the opposite arm over and place on top of your other hand. Use the top hand to pull up while you resist and stretch down. This resistance helps to create a better stretch.

Hold the stretch for at least 3 counts on each side. Do 4 to 5 total repetitions.

Reverse Wrist Stretch

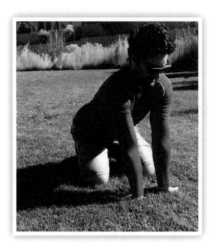

■ **Benefits:**

Stretches the wrists and fingers, helping to relieve tension and pain.

■ **How-To:**

Kneeling on the ground, bring your hands in front of your knees with the palms down and the fingers pointing back towards you. Gently press the heel of the hands down and pull the hips back to increase the stretch.

On The Ground Shoulder Roll

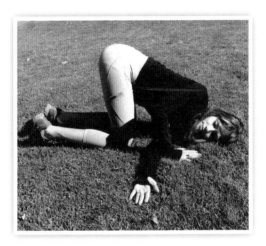

■ Benefits:

Stretches hard-to-reach spots in the shoulders and upper back.

■ How-To:

Come onto all fours. Take one hand under the body and reach as far as you can on the ground with the palm up bringing the side of the head down so that the temple and ear touch the ground. Using your other arm, push back to deepen the stretch while you continue to reach the bottom hand as far as possible.

Gorilla Stretch

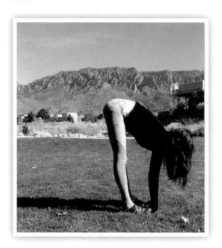

■ Benefits:

Stretches the entire back body, especially the backs of the legs and the area between the shoulder blades, and relieves the wrists and fingers of discomfort.

■ How-To:

Stand with your feet hip-width apart. Fold forward, bending the knees if necessary, to bring your hands to your feet. Slide your hands palms up under the soles of your feet so that your toes are touching the crease of your wrist. Rock forward to bring more weight into the ball of your foot providing a better stretch for your upper back and wrists. If you are barefoot, you can move the toes up and down to massage the wrists.

Legs Crossed Forward Fold

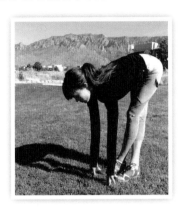

■ Benefits:

This alternate to just simply touching your toes stretches a different part of the leg, especially the iliotibial band which connects the hip joint to the knee and is a common source of pain in the outer knee due to inflammation. Crossing your legs when touching your toes strengthens and stretches the muscles of the hip that connect to the knee, helping to prevent and ease pain.

■ How-To:

Stand with your feet together. Cross one leg over the other, bringing the feet together in one line. Fold forward trying to touch your toes and place your hands either on the ground or on any part of your legs except for the knee joint. As you bend forward, engage the front of the legs by lifting the kneecaps. Contracting the front muscles of the legs allows you to stretch the back of the legs deeper.

Standing Shoulder Twist

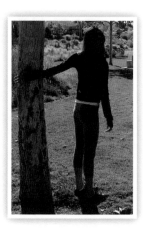

■ Benefits:

Stretches deep into the muscles of the shoulders and upper back. Because of the tendency to slouch forward throughout the day, this pose is essential in order to strengthen and loosen the muscles of the upper back and shoulders while improving posture. For this stretch you will need some sort of sturdy vertical object, such as a wall, tree, pole, or even another person.

■ How-To:

Stand close enough to a vertical surface so that one side of your body is either flush to it (like if you are using a wall) or so that your feet are in line with it and a foot or so in front. Extend your arm back so that the palm of your hand can touch the surface, thumb on top. Deepen the stretch by pressing your hand into the surface as you twist away from it.

Standing Ninety Degree Stretch

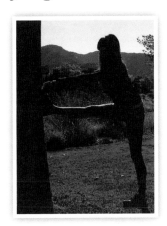

■ Benefits:

Creates a deep stretch in the back of the leg while strengthening the muscles that surround the hip. Working on balance is also great for the mind.

■ How-To:

Stand in front of a sturdy flat surface at a distance so that you can place the sole of your foot on it while keeping your leg parallel to the floor. If your leg cannot reach high enough to make a ninety-degree angle, lift it as high as you can. You do not want to lift your leg higher than a ninety-degree angle. Since your goal is to stretch the back of the lifted leg, engage the front of the leg by lifting the kneecap. Also make sure that the leg you are standing on is stable and straight. Reach forward for the lifted foot, keeping the back as straight as possible.

Tree Stretch

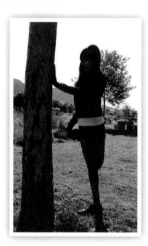 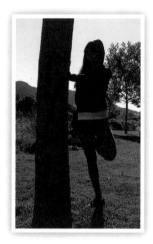

■ Benefits:

Strengthens the muscles of the legs and improves flexibility of the hips, which helps to relieve low back discomfort and reduce the risk of injury.

■ How-To:

It is a good idea to start by using a wall or tree for balance but you can do this pose without as well.

Stand tall with your feet together. Lift one foot up and bring the sole of the foot to the hip crease. Keep the leg that you are standing on straight and sturdy. To work on opening the hip, draw the knee of the lifted leg back as you press the hips forward. Try to get both knees in one even plane.

Heel To Butt Stretch

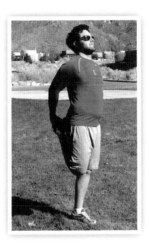

■ **Benefits:**

Stretches the front of the upper leg and hip flexor while improving balance, which is good for the brain and great for injury prevention.

■ **How-To:**

It is a good idea to start using a wall or tree for balance but you can do this pose without as well.

Stand tall with your feet together. Lift one foot off the ground, bending the knee and bringing your heel to your butt. Keep both knees together as much as possible. To increase the stretch pull the foot closer to your butt with your hands while you simultaneously kick the foot back into your hand.

Standing Calf Stretch

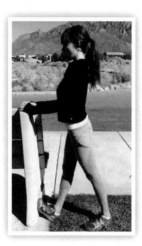

■ Benefits:

This pose is very straightforward, but it is one of the best ways to, as the name implies, stretch the calf muscle at the back of your leg.

■ How-To:

Find a surface that you can press your foot into, such as a wall, a tree, or a curb.

Stand so that you can place the sole of the foot onto the surface while keeping the heel on the ground. Intensify the stretch by pressing your foot firmly against the surface and placing more of the sole of your foot onto the surface.

Standing Total Leg Stretch

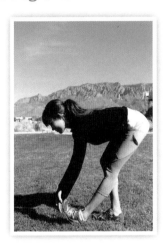

■ Benefits:

This stretch targets many of the muscles in the back of the leg, including ones that can be tough to get to.

■ How-To:

Stand with your feet together. Step one foot slightly forward while bending the knee of the other leg just slightly. Keep the front leg straight and extended with the kneecap lifted. Lift the toes of the front leg and reach down with both hands. Use your arms to pull yourself down over the front leg as you simultaneously pull your hips back.

Easy Backbend

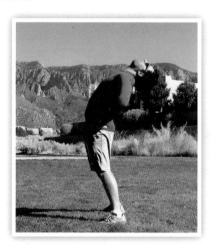

■ Benefits:

This stretch helps to counteract a day's worth of sitting. It helps to elongate the entire spine while also opening the chest. Opening the chest helps to increase lung capacity and refreshes the body and mind.

■ How-To:

Stand tall with your feet together. To make this stretch easier you can stand with the feet hip-width apart. Bring your hands to your hips or onto your low back. Push your hips forward as you start to bend backwards. The key to bending back further is being able to relax the muscles around the spine and spinning the inner thighs back to help create more space for the spine.

Open Arm Swing

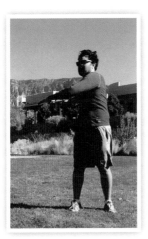 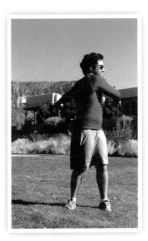

■ Benefits:

This dynamic stretch increases the range of motion in the shoulders and back while also relieving tension in both areas.

■ How-To:

Stand with your feet hip width apart. Raise your arms so that they are perpendicular to your body, but keep the shoulders relaxed to allow for maximum stretching. Twisting from the hips start to swing one arm behind you allowing the torso to follow with it. Twist from side to side and use the momentum to get deeper into the stretch each time.

Arm Across Chest

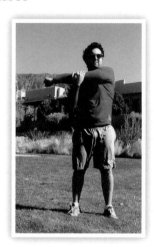

■ **Benefits:**

Uses resistance to stretch and increase the flexibility of the upper arm and shoulder.

■ **How-To:**

Bring one arm across the body at shoulder height with the elbow slightly bent. Use your other hand to press the upper arm in towards your chest. Simultaneously, draw the shoulder of the arm that is being stretched back into its socket. The resistance created by doing this will help to increase the flexibility of your shoulder faster than just simply pressing the arm into the chest.

Eagle Arms

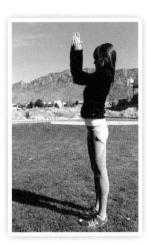

■ **Benefits:**

This stretch releases tension in the upper back, particularly the rhomboids, while helping to relieve pain and heal scar tissue in the wrists and elbows.

■ **How-To:**

Bring your arms straight out in front of you with the palms facing in. Pull the arms back in towards the shoulder socket. Cross one arm over the other at the elbow and bend both elbows. Bring the arm that is on top under the wrist of the opposite arm. Join the palms of the hands together or interlace the fingers. To maximize the benefits of this pose, lift the elbows up and press the forearms forward.

Knee Down Lunge

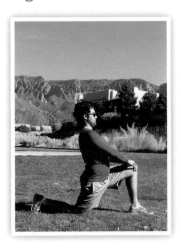

■ Benefits:

Refines balance while stretching and strengthening the muscles surrounding the hips.

■ How-To:

Stand tall with your feet hip width apart. Take a big step forward with one of your feet and bring the knee of the back leg down to the ground. Adjust your stance so that you feel a stretch in the hip of the back leg and so that the knee of your front leg is directly over the ankle. Press back into the foot of the back leg as you simultaneously lower your hips down closer to the ground.

Easy Half Splits

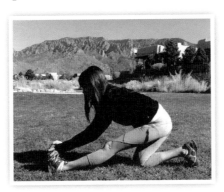

■ **Benefits:**

Creates an intense stretch in the back of the leg while also stretching the sole of the foot, which can provide relief from foot cramps and plantar fasciitis. You can also work on improving your balance in this stretch.

■ **How-To:**

Come into a low squat so that you are close, but not quite sitting on your heels. Extend one leg straight out in front of you and flex the foot back towards your face. In order to stretch the sole and arches of the other foot, keep the toes tucked with the weight in the ball of the foot. Reach forward with one or both hands (both hands will challenge your balance) and grab the foot of the extended leg. Pull your hips back as you reach forward, getting as low as you can to the extended leg.

Down Dog Stretch

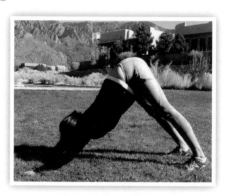

■ Benefits:

This stretch helps to increase the range of motion in your shoulders while simultaneously strengthening your upper body. It also stretches the backs of your legs, primarily the hamstrings and the calves.

■ How-To:

Come down to all fours. Straighten the legs and lift the hips back and up. Your hands should be shoulder-width apart with the fingers spread wide. Press your torso back so that your ears are next to your biceps or upper arms. Your feet should be hip-width apart with the heels directly behind your toes. Try to press your heels down towards the ground and slightly lift the toes to help stretch your calves. To better stretch your hamstrings, lift the kneecaps and engage the fronts of your thighs.

Three-Leg Down Dog

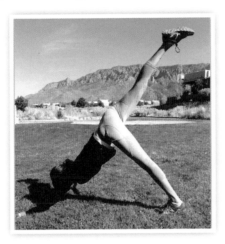

■ Benefits:

Similar to Down Dog, this stretch will strengthen your upper body and improve the flexibility of your shoulders. The lifted leg helps to increase the strength and flexibility of the hip flexor while the leg on the ground still receives a beneficial stretch in the hamstring and calf.

■ How-To:

Come down to all fours. Straighten the legs and lift the hips back and up. Your hands should be shoulder-width apart with the fingers spread wide. Press your torso back so that your ears are next to your biceps or upper arms. Your feet should be hip-width apart with the heels directly behind your toes. Try to press your heels down towards the ground and slightly lift the toes to help stretch your calves. To better stretch your hamstrings, lift the kneecaps and engage the fronts of your thighs.

Lift one of your legs straight up and back, doing your best to keep both hips in one even line. As you lift your leg higher continue to press down through the heel of the foot on the ground.

Pigeon Stretch

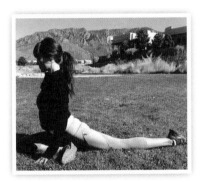

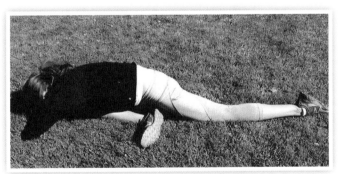

■ **Benefits:**

Deeply stretches the hips, creating more flexibility and relieving built-up tension. Opening the hips is beneficial because it reduces pain and discomfort in the low back.

■ How-To:

Come down to all fours. Slide your right knee forwards toward your right wrist. Lower the hips down to the ground and extend your back leg out behind you as if you were going to do the splits. To get more of a stretch in your outer hip move the foot of the front leg forward.

You can also refine this stretch by folding forward over your front leg and bringing your head down to the ground. In order to get deeper into the muscles of the hips, try to relax as much as possible. If your muscles are tense it is, obviously, more difficult to stretch them.

Super Pigeon Stretch

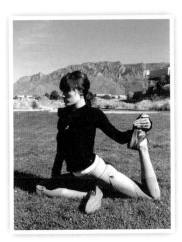

■ **Benefits:**

Like Pigeon, this stretch improves flexibility of the hips, but also stretches the quadriceps.

■ **How-To:**

Come down to all fours. Slide your right knee forwards toward your right wrist. Lower the hips down to the ground and extend your back leg out behind you as if you were going to do the splits. To get more of a stretch in your outer hip move the foot of the front leg forward. Bend the back leg at the knee and reach back with the same arm to grab the ankle. To create resistance, press your hips forward and down as you kick the foot of the back leg back into your hand.

Runner's Lunge

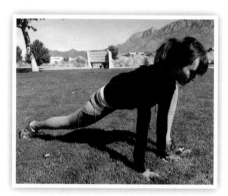

■ **Benefits:**

This stretch works on improving the flexibility of the hips, hamstrings, and thighs.

■ **How-To:**

Come down to all fours. Extend one leg straight back behind you, keeping the knee lifted of the ground and weight in the ball of the foot. Step the front foot forward so that it is even with your hands. Both hands should be placed on the inside of the front foot. Press the hips down and keep the back straight. To create resistance, continue pressing back through the extended back leg and into the ball of the foot.

Super Lunge Twist

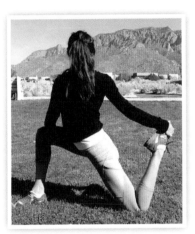

■ Benefits:

Stretches the muscles of the hip and the quadriceps while opening the chest and shoulders. The twisted position of this stretch helps to increase flexibility of the spine.

■ How-To:

Come down to all fours. Step the right foot forward by your right hand. Press yourself up so you are sitting up tall. Keep the left knee down on the ground. Bring your left forearm to your right thigh and reach back with your right arm. Bend the back knee to bring your heel in towards the body. Grab your left foot with your right hand. Kick your left foot back into the hand as much as possible to help you maintain your balance and get a deeper stretch.

Playful Puppy Stretch

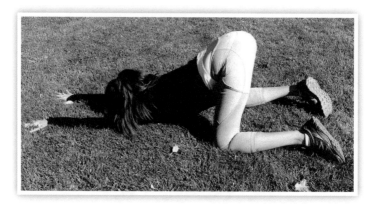

■ Benefits:

Improves flexibility of the total spine and shoulders. Relieves tension in the area of the upper back between the shoulder blades.

■ How-To:

Come down to all fours. Walk the arms forward until you can bring your head all the way to the ground. Adjust your legs if necessary so that your knees stay right under your hips. To get the maximum stretch in this position continue walking your hands forward as much as possible while simultaneously pulling your hips back. The traction that is created by doing so helps to lengthen spine while opening the shoulders at the same time.

Easy Seated Twist

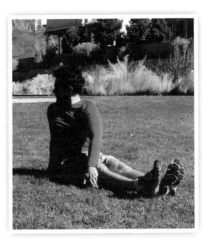

■ Benefits:

Gently stretches the back, helping to increase flexibility and decrease discomfort created from sitting for long periods of time.

■ How-To:

Sit on the ground with your legs extended straight out in front of you. Keep the legs together as you bring the left hand to the outside of the right leg. Place your right hand on the ground at the base of spine to help you twist further while maintaining a long spine. As you inhale, use the right hand to sit up straighter. As you exhale, use the left hand to help you twist around further.

Seated Spine Twist

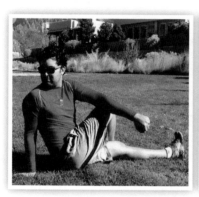 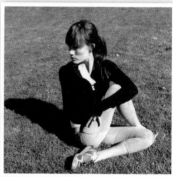

■ Benefits:

This stretch does wonders for relieving pain in the lower back while also helping to increase the range of motion of the shoulders and upper back. It also stretches the sides of the hips and the gluteus muscles.

■ How-To:

Sit on the ground with your legs extended straight in front of you. Cross the right leg over the left keeping the knee bent and in close to the body. You can opt to either leave the left leg extended on the ground or you can bend the left knee and bring the heel of the foot to the outside of the right hip. Take your left arm up and over the right knee, gently pressing into the knee to help you twist back. Place the right hand on the ground at the base of the spine and use it to help you sit up tall.

Seated Forward Fold

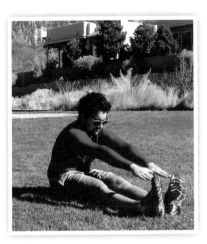

■ **Benefits:**

This stretch helps to calm and soothe the mind while lowering blood pressure and providing an intense opening for the entire back of the body.

■ **How-To:**

Sit on the ground with legs extended straight out in front of you. Flex the feet back towards the face and press the thighbones firmly down into the ground. Sit up as tall as possible and squeeze the shoulder blades together slightly to help keep the back straight and engaged. Keeping a straight spine, start to slowly fold forward from the hips, reaching for your toes. The stretch comes from folding at the hip crease and flexing the legs, not from getting as low as possible.

One-Legged Seated Fold

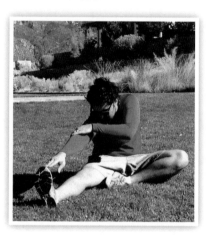

■ Benefits:

It helps to stretch the muscles of the back, hamstrings, and gluteus muscles. Forward folds such as this also help to calm the mind and lower blood pressure.

■ How-To:

Sit with your legs extended straight out in front of you. Bend one knee to bring the sole of the foot to the inside of the other leg's upper thigh. Press your hands into the ground on either side of the body to help lengthen the spine before you fold. Keeping the muscles of the upper back engaged, begin to fold over the extended leg. Fold from the hip creases rather than rounding the spine. Energetically pull the heel of the extended leg towards you while simultaneously engaging the quadriceps and pressing the thighbone down.

One-Legged Seated Twist

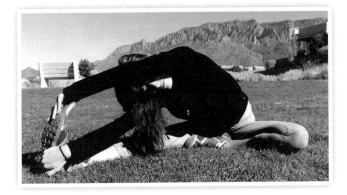

■ **Benefits:**

Stretches the back of the extended leg while opening the shoulders and chest. Twisting the spine helps to increase range of motion and flexibility in the back.

■ **How-To:**

Sit with your legs extended straight out in front of you. Bend one knee to bring the sole of the foot to the inside of the other leg's upper thigh. Press your hands into the ground on either side of the body to help lengthen the spine. Lean towards the extended leg, pressing the top shoulder back and the bottom shoulder under to open the chest and shoulders. Use the bottom hand to grab onto the arch of the foot. The top arm should extend over the head and towards the foot, possibly holding onto the toes of the extended leg. Continue to twist your upper body up towards the sky while simultaneously lowering the body down closer to the leg.

Cow Face Leg Stretch

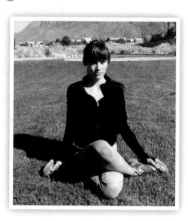

■ Benefits:

This stretch helps to improve flexibility of the lower back and hips. It also relieves tension by stimulating the knee and ankle joints. It is very beneficial for people who suffer from constant backaches or sciatica pain.

■ How-To:

Sit on the ground with your legs extended straight in front of you. Cross one leg on top of the other bringing the foot as close as you can to the opposite hip. Lower the knee down towards the ground. Bend the knee of the bottom leg and bring the foot as close as you can to the opposite hip. Bring that knee down on top of the bottom knee. Use your hands at either side of the body to help you sit straight. Continue to intensify this stretch by pressing the knees down and pulling the hip bones back.

Hero's Stretch

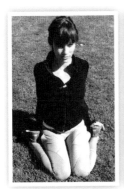
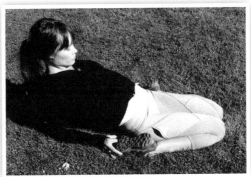

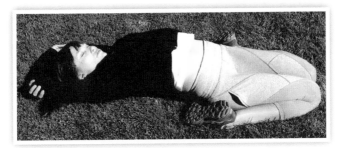

■ Benefits:

Deeply stretches the thigh muscles while increasing flexibility and health in the knee and ankle joints. Depending on the variation, this stretch also opens the chest.

■ How-To:

Kneel on the ground and sit back on your heels. Bring the ankles and feet out from under the body and place on either side of the hips, sitting down on the rougnd. The soles of the feet face up and the toes point straight back. Try to keep your knees as close together as possible. If this position is painful you can place something under your seat to lift you up and take pressure off of the knees and ankles.

To open the chest and get a deeper stretch in the thighs, reach the hands behind your body and bring the forearms down to the ground. Squeeze the shoulder blades together and lift the chest up.

To get even deeper, lower your torso all the way down to the ground. If your knees come off the ground as you do this go back to the forearms. If you can comfortably lie down, reach the arms overhead and grab opposite elbows to continue to open the chest and shoulders.

Seated Hip Opener

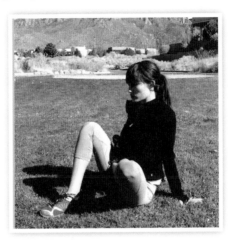

■ Benefits:

Increases the mobility of the hip joint while stretching the gluteus muscle and relieving discomfort in the lower back.

■ How-To:

Sit on the ground with your legs extended straight in front of you. Place your left foot on top of the right thigh. Begin to bend the right knee, sliding the foot back towards your body until you feel a good stretch in the left hip. Place your hands behind your body to help to keep you sitting up straight. To increase the stretch, continue bringing the right foot closer towards the body and pressing the left knee away from your body.

Knees To Chest

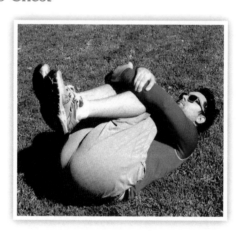

■ Benefits:

This stretch relieves pain in the lower back while also improving the functioning of the digestive organs.

■ How-To:

Lie down flat on your back with your legs extended straight in front of you. Bend the knees and bring them towards your chest keeping the legs together. Grab opposite elbows, forearms, or interlace your fingers and squeeze the knees together and towards your body. At the same time, press your shoulders and tailbone down into the ground, working to get the entire spine flat on the ground.

Thread The Needle

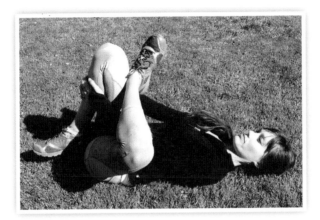

■ Benefits:

This stretch releases the gluteus muscles while stretching the muscles of the hips. If done consistently, this stretch can relieve sciatic pain as well.

■ How-To:

Lie down flat on your back with your legs extended straight in front of you. Begin to bend the knees and place the ankle of the left foot onto the thigh of the right leg. Bend the right knee and bring the foot in as close as you can to your body. Interlace your fingers around the shin of the right leg by threading your left arm in between the opening made with your legs. Your right hand should reach around the outside of the right leg. Gently pull the right knee towards your body as you press the left knee away.

Supine One Leg Pull

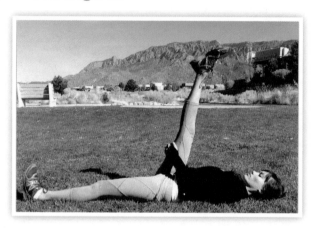

■ Benefits:

Increases flexibility of the hips while stretching the back of the lifted leg.

■ How-To:

Lie down flat on your back with your legs extended straight in front of you. Begin to lift one of your legs into the air. Try to keep both legs straight and the bottom leg on the ground. Grab onto the back of the thigh of the lifted leg and gently pull it closer towards your body. If you cannot keep the shoulders on the ground, use something like a dog leash around the lifted leg so that you can pull on the leash to bring your leg closer while keeping your spine flat along the ground. To create resistance in this stretch, use your arms to pull your leg in as your leg pushes away from your body.

Total Twist

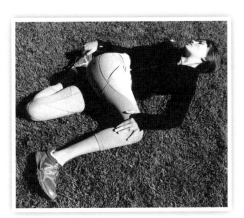

■ Benefits:

This stretch is the total deal because of its ability to stretch the back, shoulders, hips, and quadriceps at the same time. It is one of the best stretches to do if you suffer from severe lower back pain or even just mild discomfort.

■ How-To:

Lie flat on your back with your legs extended straight in front of you. Bring the right knee in towards your chest while keeping the left leg extended along the ground. Bring the right knee over the body allowing the foot and knee to come down towards the ground. Use your left hand to gently press the knee down so that you can increase the twist. Bend the knee of the left leg and bring the heel back towards your body. With your right hand, grab onto the foot and pull to stretch the quadriceps.

Extended Child's Pose

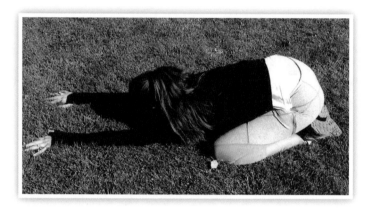

■ **Benefits:**

This stretch is great for helping your body relax while simultaneously stretching the quadriceps, lengthening the spine, and opening the hips. It also helps to relieve lower back discomfort. This stretch is a great place to hang out for a while to calm your mind and distress.

■ **How-To:**

Kneel on the ground. Separate your knees at least hip distance but keep your toes together and the tops of your feet on the ground. Fold forward in between your knees, reaching the arms straight out in front of you. Bring your forehead down onto the ground and you hips back to your heels. To create traction to lengthen the spine, continue to walk your hands forward while pulling your hips back down towards your heels.

HOW IS YOGA DIFFERENT FROM STRETCHING?

People often wonder how stretching is different from yoga because the two often feel and look so similar. One of the major differences (it's major but subtle) is the attention to breath that is cultivated during yoga practice that is often ignored while stretching. There are a lot of benefits that come from learning to focus on your breath while entering challenging stretches, including learning how to effectively deal with stress and how to be present for each moment of your day.

There are also many different styles of yoga that perform the stretches differently. Certain types, such as restorative classes, hold a stretch for a really long time (like 10 to 15 minutes each), doing only 4 or 5 in an hour-long class. Others, like Vinyasa, flow from one pose to the next, creating an intense cardio workout while stretching. And then there are power types of yoga, such as Ashtanga, that performs stretches while incorporating major muscle strengthening exercises.

Stretching, whether done on its own or in a yoga class, is always beneficial to your body, keeping it flexible, youthful, and free of pain.

If you are interested in learning more about yoga, here are a few of my other books that help to explain specific yoga poses, the benefits of meditation, and how learning to breathe correctly can change your life.

Books on Yoga

- Yoga Poses For The New Yogi: 37 Wickedly Effective Yoga Postures To Transform Your Day
- Christian Yoga: A Daily Christian Meditation Guide For Your Practice
- Super Hot Yoga Beach Body: Yoga Fitness Secrets To Supercharge Your Sex Appeal

Books on Meditation

- Chakra Meditation: A Down To Earth Guide For Healing Chakras and Balancing Chakras
- How To Meditate Like Buddha: Beginner's Meditation Guide

Books on Breathing

- Keep Calm and Breathe: 10 Deep Breathing Techniques To Bring Awareness, Relieve Stress, Reduce Anxiety, and Change Your Life Forever

STRETCH INDEX

Shoulders

- Elbow Behind Head
- Elbow Behind Head Bind
- Wide Legged Forward Fold
- Wide Legged Twist
- Wide Legged Forward Bend With Clasp
- Compass Twist
- On The Ground Shoulder Roll
- Standing Shoulder Twist
- Open Arm Swing
- Arm Across Chest
- Down Dog Stretch
- Three-Leg Down Dog
- Super Lunge Twist
- Playful Puppy Stretch
- Seated Spine Twist
- One-Legged Seated Twist
- Total Twist

Back

- Wide Legged Forward Fold
- Wide Legged Twist
- Wide Legged Lunge
- On The Ground Shoulder Roll
- Gorilla Stretch
- Standing Shoulder Twist
- Easy Backbend
- Open Arm Swing
- Eagle Arms
- Super Lunge Twist
- Playful Puppy Stretch
- Easy Seated Twist
- Seated Spine Twist
- Seated Forward Fold
- One-Legged Seated Fold
- One-Legged Seated Twist
- Cow Face Leg Stretch
- Seated Hip Opener
- Knees To Chest
- Total Twist
- Extended Child's Pose

Hips

- Wide Legged Lunge
- Legs Crossed Forward Fold
- Tree Stretch
- Heel To Butt Stretch
- Knee Down Lunge
- Three-Leg Down Dog
- Pigeon Stretch

- Super Pigeon Stretch
- Runner's Lunge
- Super Lunge Twist
- Seated Spine Twist
- Cow Face Leg Stretch
- Seated Hip Opener
- Thread The Needle
- Supine One Leg Pull
- Total Twist

Quadriceps

- Heel To Butt Stretch
- Super Pigeon Stretch
- Runner's Lunge
- Super Lunge Twist
- Hero's Stretch
- Total Twist
- Extended Child's Pose

Hamstrings

- Wide Legged Forward Fold
- Wide Legged Twist
- Wide Legged Forward Bend With Clasp
- Compass Twist
- Gorilla Stretch
- Legs Crossed Forward Fold
- Standing Ninety Degree Stretch
- Standing Total Leg Stretch
- Easy Half Splits
- Down Dog Stretch
- Three-Leg Down Dog
- Runner's Lunge

- Seated Forward Fold
- One-Legged Seated Fold
- One-Legged Seated Twist
- Supine One Leg Pull

Calves

- Gorilla Stretch
- Standing Calf Stretch
- Standing Total Leg Stretch
- Down Dog Stretch
- Three-Leg Down Dog
- Seated Forward Fold
- One-Legged Seated Fold
- One-Legged Seated Twist

Wrists

- Twisted Wrist Roll
- Reverse Wrist Stretch
- Gorilla Stretch
- Eagle Arms

ABOUT THE AUTHOR

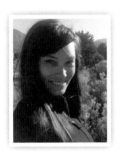 **Julie Schoen** is an author, yoga instructor, former model, teacher, and co-founder of the company Little Pearl Publishing, dedicated to bringing the world "little pearls" of wisdom.

Over the past six years, Julie Schoen has dedicated her life to pursuing knowledge and sharing it through her writing and teaching. In 2005, she was in a hit-and-run car accident, leaving her with serious injuries to her head and spine. After consulting numerous physical therapists and chiropractors, Schoen turned to yoga and meditation to heal her body and spirit. During the long healing process from this accident, she developed a new gratefulness for life's opportunities and takes advantage of each one that she is given.

As an experienced teacher and yoga instructor, Schoen has traveled the world studying with and absorbing the wisdom of each person she meets. A devoted wife and mom, she is thankful for the opportunity to make a living writing, teaching, and traveling, while still being present for every moment of her life.

Discover More Great Books At
Little Pearl Publishing
(littlepearlpublishing.com)

Made in the USA
Lexington, KY
22 May 2014